Table of Contents

Tips Related to Office/Admin Staff – The Backbone of Your Home Care Business

Tips Related to Recruiting, Retaining, and Managing Caregivers

Tips Related to Providing Good Client Care

Tips Related to Your Own Leadership, Time Management, and Self-Care

Tips to Grow Your Home Care Business

Challenges

Startup and ongoing costs

Finding and keeping quality staff

Closing the communication gap with hospitals and medical providers

Confusion with "Home Care vs Home Health Care; Medical vs Non-Medical"

Promising growth, daunting challenges

INRODUCTION

What do you think about when you think about the elderly? Will you be like them when you grow old? Why does it seem that they react and perceive the world around them so differently from you and I? Why is it sometimes so difficult to predict and understand how they will respond to the people around them and to their surroundings?

In order to understand the elderly better, it is important to understand how some of the changes they experience as they age affect them. Here are some of the key areas of change which affect us all as we grow older.

Physical Changes

As we grow older, bone loss, arthritis and other health issues begin to make it harder for us to participate in some activities. Other changes such as the loss of teeth may make it difficult for us to enjoy simple activities such as eating. Physical deterioration begins to reduce the types of things which we can do and enjoy.

Sensory Losses

From about the age of 40 onwards, most people start to experience some form of decline in visual ability. Some develop cataracts or glaucoma which require treatment or even surgery. Losing the ability to see is frightening and affects a person's confidence in performing daily tasks.

Hearing loss is another common problem. Not all adjust

well to it and this difficulty can result in arguments and miscommunication between the elderly and the young and an acute sense of isolation.

The ability to detect different tastes also declines with age. This is why food may seem bland to the older person.

The Cardiovascular and Nervous System

With age, changes take place in the blood vessels that increase the risk of coronary heart disease and hypertension. An older person also takes longer to respond to external stimuli. An older person crossing the road might require a longer time to do so and may not be as aware of approaching cars. Elderly people are at risk in situations such as these.

Social Roles

When a person retires, the loss of job titles, position and status may lead to grief, depression and diminished self-esteem. As children grow up and move away to start families of their own, older people experience changes not only professionally, but also personally and it may take time to adjust to new roles and expectations.

Financial Status

Without a job, a person's income is affected. Some elderly people may need to make changes to their lifestyles to match changes in their income.

Accommodation

Most elderly people do not like to move to a new house or an unfamiliar environment. They usually take a longer time to adjust to new places and people. So, if a change in residence is necessary, it is important to prepare them in advance and to take their views into consideration.

Activities and Hobbies

Whilst most people think that retirement marks the ideal time to start new hobbies and activities, you need to be aware that physical limitations may mean that the elderly may not be able to participate fully in a hobby or an activity. For elderly people in this situation, life can become even more depressing and boring.

Relationships

It is important to recognize that as their friends, relatives and spouses grow older and become ill or pass away that the elderly will still need our support for companionship, love and affection.

IMPORTANCE OF ELDERLY CARE SERVICES

Old age is a sensitive phase; elderly people need care and comfort to lead a healthy life without worries and anxiety. Lack of awareness regarding the changing behavioral patterns in elderly people at home leads to abuse of them by their kin.

Birth, childhood, adolescence, adulthood and old age are the most crucial stages in a man's life. All these stages have their very own issues and troubles. As each level passes the physical strength deteriorates as well as the mental stability lessens. Since age progresses, various medical issues happen, some of the particular known diseases usually are blood pressure, diabetes, heart failure issues, arthritis, cancer malignancy, joint pains, tuberculosis, as well as kidney infections.

It's just not disease that affects old age; there are various other issues that govern the downfall of the health of the old people. One of the main issues is the negligence from the younger generation. Old people need supervision, the laxity to understand the needs and worries of elders make them appear strangers to the younger generation, who later regard them as a burden.

Old people are subject to abuse from family members over property dispute, some of them are even forced to sell their belongings and live in penury till death. Many of them are too scared to express themselves or fear being humiliated by their loved ones.

Elders desire a life with good health, dignity, economic independence and finally a peaceful death. They long for care, love and affection. Understanding their needs and concerns, will ensure their good health. Lending an emotional support to the elders keep them jovial, which is inevitably the ideal way to live a healthy life. However, for many people, providing care and attention to elders is not possible due to work priorities.

Elders suffering from cognitive challenges' undergo serious personality changes; at this point they need care and attention. When they are left unattended, most of them are gripped with overwhelming feelings of dejection, purposelessness; some of them even turn violent. Regardless of the fact that many of us know that aging is a natural progression and it has its own shortcoming, most of us tend to ignore this and resort to an unruly approach.

HOME CARE

The World Health Organization states that, "Home care can be defined as an array of health and social support services provided to clients in their own residence. Such coordinated services may prevent, delay, or be a substitute for temporary or long-term institutional care."

Palliative home care is the care provided by professionals to people in their own homes with the ultimate goal of not only contributing to their life quality and functional health status, but also to replace hospital care with care in the home for societal reasons. Home care covers a wide range of activities, from preventive visits to end-of-life care.

Home Care allows our elderly community to live more independently and continue to enjoy the lives they've built at home. Elderly care services allow older adults to continue living their day-to-day lives as they always have. Therefore, a little help with those tasks that become challenging with age will make it easier. As life expectancy grows, these residential care services are becoming a necessary part of our communities. Home care services help ensure that our elderly family members continue to thrive throughout their lives.

Home Care Services:

There are several distinct types of Home Care services accessible, each with certain advantages. Home care services can help seniors live more independently in their houses longer. They may also assist caregivers who are fatigued by their duties.

- Personal Care: This home care service includes bathing, dressing, and grooming. It also includes assistance with toileting and incontinence care.
- Homemaker Services: This type of home caregiving task include laundry, grocery shopping, meal preparation, and light housekeeping. Hence, it can help seniors stay home longer by providing necessary support with everyday tasks.
- Companionship Services: This home care provides companion care for seniors who may be lonely or isolated. Hence, it can provide social interaction and stimulation and help seniors avoid depression and anxiety.
- Respite Care: This home care provides temporary relief for caregivers who feel overwhelmed or burnt out. Therefore, Home Care of this sort is ideal for caregivers who need a temporary break from their care schedule. It can give caregivers a chance to relax and get support when they need it most.
- Home Health aide Services: Home health care is a form of skilled health care that includes specialized registered nurses services, such as physical and occupational therapy, speech-language therapy, and other medically cared services. Home health nurses give and assist with delivering treatment and therapy ordered by your doctor.

BENEFITS OF HOME CARE

There are many benefits of home care, both for seniors and caregivers. Without a doubt, there are many proven benefits of Home Care, and some of them are:

- Seniors can maintain their independence and live in their own homes for longer periods.
- Caregivers can provide much-needed support and assistance with activities of daily living.
- Home care can provide social interaction and companionship for seniors who may be lonely or isolated.
- Agency caregivers can give a break for family caregivers and provide respite care during times of stress.
- Home care is often more affordable than other forms of long-term care.

HOME HEALTHCARE MARKET

The global home healthcare market size was valued at USD 362.1 billion in 2022 and is expected to expand at a compound annual growth rate (CAGR) of 7.96% from 2023 to 2030. The growing geriatric population and rising incidence of target diseases such as dementia and Alzheimer's as well as orthopedic diseases are factors expected to fuel market growth. Increasing treatment cost is one of the prime concerns for governments and health organizations, and hence they are striving to curb healthcare costs. Home healthcare is a cost-efficient alternative to an expensive hospital stay.

For instance, as per a report by The Commonwealth Fund, "hospital at home" programs enable patients to receive acute care at home with fewer complications and over 30% reduction in the cost of care. This helps ensure patient comfort and is projected to serve as a high impact rendering driver of the market. Advancements in medicine have led to a shift from communicable to noncommunicable diseases in developing countries. Sedentary lifestyle and high consumption of alcohol are factors responsible for increase in the prevalence of lifestyle diseases. Growing incidence of target diseases requiring long-term care, such as Alzheimer's disease and dementia, is expected to drive the market during the forecast period.

Furthermore, awareness about home care services and devices for such conditions is increasing. Availability of portable devices such as heart rate monitors, respiratory aids, and blood glucose monitors has improved the efficiency and effectiveness of home care for lifestyle diseases. Value-based healthcare is another major factor contributing to the market. In most of the developed and developing nations, the central government is offering either partial or complete coverage for the in-home services. In the U.S., Medicare reimbursements are highly favorable in providing value-based healthcare for improved patient outcomes at a low cost. Thus, in-home care has become a modality of choice for treatment.

WHY YOU SHOULD INVEST IN A HOME CARE BUSINESS

Besides a booming elderly population, there are many reasons for small business owners in Canada to invest in a home care business, including the following:

You'll feel good about doing it

When you choose to work with a vulnerable population, like children, or the elderly, you are inevitably making a difference in their everyday quality of life. Something as simple as having a quick conversation with your patients every morning or taking the time to get to know them on a personal level can make all the difference in the world for those living in a long-term care facility, especially if they have no family of their own, or can't see their family as much as they'd like.

Demand for home care is at an all-time high

As statistics show, Canada's ageing population is only going up. The demand for home care services for seniors is increasing, especially as the debate around how COVID-19 is managed in private healthcare facilities continues to be a topic of concern. Many seniors do not want to enter a long-term care facility because they want to hold on to their homes, which is another reason that personal care done out of a home is becoming so popular.

FAQS ABOUT STARTING A SENIOR HOME CARE BUSINESS

America is aging fast. There are now almost 50 million senior citizens over 65 in the U.S, and that number is expected to double in just a few years. As seniors age, especially in their 70s and 80s, they need more help at home doing tasks most younger folks take for granted, which means a growing need for a senior home care business in every community, large or small.

Because of their age and health issues, many seniors are homebound or less mobile, and need a bit of help at home with some of the routine tasks that used to be so easy for them, like meal preparation, light housekeeping, shopping and errands. As little as two hours a day of help can make a big difference – enabling seniors to remain in their own homes – which is what 90% of them want. At home, they have familiar surroundings, privacy and independence.

Because of this senior population boom, the demand for senior services has grown swiftly to keep pace. One of the best senior service businesses is a senior home care business. It's a profitable and satisfying way to help others and make good money doing it. If you're not familiar with it, you may have some questions before you're ready to get started. Here are some of the most commonly asked questions:

What does a senior home care provider do?

Most senior home care clients are between 65 and 95 years old, living in their own home, who just need help with daily living activities, such as laundry, meal preparation, housekeeping and medication reminders. A home care provider helps them live at home by taking care of these tasks, and also provide companionship by listening to their clients, reading a book to them or playing cards.

How much are senior home caregivers paid?

There is a big difference in the pay for caregivers who work for a home care agency and those who have their own independent home care service. For example, an agency might charge the client $24 an hour, but only pay the caregiver $12 an hour. That's why it's best to be an independent caregiver, with your own business name, so you can get the best rates in your area. If you're getting paid $12 an hour, you'll make just $24,000 a year.As an independent caregiver, doing the same work, you'll be able to charge $24, and make $48,000 a year. Which would you rather earn – $24,000 or $48,000?

Who hires senior home care providers?

Senior care professionals, such as discharge planners at local hospitals and assisted-living facilities are always looking for capable, reliable home caregivers. Adult children of seniors who need in-home care are a prime source of new clients as well. Many of them use the internet to search for a caregiver, so it's a good idea to register with one or more of the online care provider referral services, such as eldercare link.com.

What accounts for the rapid growth of the business?

Home care services are the fastest growing part of the entire health care industry in America. In fact, the U.S. Department of Labor says non-medical home caregivers are the most in-demand job now, and likely for the next two decades. There are two reasons for this demand. First, medical advances have made it possible for people to be cared for at home rather than in a hospital or nursing home. Second, increasing costs of health care have created a growing demand for more affordable in-home care.

What's the difference between in-home health care and non-medical home care?

In home health care requires medically trained health care workers, such as nurses. Non-medical care involves only the tasks that do not require medical training. For example, a non-medical home care provider can remind a client to take their medications, but can not administer the medications.

Can I work part-time?

Yes, in most instances you can. You can tailor your work schedule to work as much or as little as you want to allow you time for other things, such as family responsibilities. Most non-medical home care clients only require 3-4 hours per day, so you could work half-days, for example.

Is it expensive to get started?

Not at all. All you really need is transportation, which in most areas means a reliable vehicle. In many cities, it's easier to use public transportation because of parking and traffic issues. Of course, you'll need a cellphone to stay in touch with clients and prospects. Any other items needed by a specific client would be provided by and paid for by the client or their family. When you're starting out, you'll need business cards and flyers or brochures, but that is a small expense, usually less than $300.

What if I've never done this before?

Non-medical in-home care is not rocket science, so if you have basic housekeeping skills, you'll do just fine. If you're unsure of yourself, go to work for a home care agency for a few weeks to learn what is needed to do a good job. If you're a caring person and a good listener, you'll do well.

How do I find customers?

Because there is such a demand for good home care providers, you just need to let prospects know that you are available. There are a dozen local sources of free referrals listed in my book. The best source of new clients, of course, is word of mouth from satisfied clients. When you're first starting out, leave a few business cards and flyers or brochures at the local senior center and run a free ad at Craigslist.org

Do I need any special training or a certificate?

Unless you plan to offer home health care services, which would require medical training, there are no class requirements or certification. In some areas, the Red Cross offers home care classes, and a few community colleges also have programs. Although there are currently no formal training requirements, you should try to learn more about your work, and perhaps even consider getting a CNA certificate. That training will help you do a better job for clients, and allow you to charge a bit more for your services.

As a home care provider, you can earn a solid, dependable income regardless of what the job market is doing. It's as close to recession-proof as it gets, as seniors continue to get older and require in-home caregivers.

HOW TO START A HOME HEALTH CARE BUSINESS SUCCESSFULLY

As the global job market continues to change rapidly and unpredictably, many people are taking this time to think about other options for the next phase of their careers. For those interested in starting their own business or purchasing a franchise, home health care makes sense. As demand continues to grow, people are increasingly seeing the opportunity in-home health care businesses. If your idea of fulfillment is helping family or friends age more comfortably, there's a real opportunity to combine purpose and profit to build an organization with heart—especially now.

As with anything, it's important to do your research.

So what's actually involved in setting up a home health care agency? Here's an executive summary of what:

- To make it legal, who should I talk to?
- What licenses do I need?
- How long does it take to get approval?
- What insurance do I need?

- How much does it really cost?

The home care business industry is growing at a rapid pace. The home care industry is rising to meet the demand. According to the Industry Market Research Report, as of 2018, the American senior care business industry revenue is expected to grow at an annualized rate of 3.3% to $92.8 billion.

Factors such as the aging population, prevalence of chronic diseases, medical professionals growing acceptance of home care, medical advancements, the longevity of life and more have contributed to significant growth of the senior home care business sector.

What Services Does a Home Health Care Business Provide?

The term home health care means providing supportive or assisted care provided by a professional caregiver or a nurse in the comfort of the patient's own home or place of living. Caregivers & nurses set up appointments and visit the client's home to provide help.

This help can be of different types ranging from companionship to medication administration. Even though home care involves medical assistance, most forms of home health care revolve around providing basic assistance like personal care, grocery assistance, and companionship.

Medical Or Non-Medical Home Health Care Business?

Choosing what kind of services to offer is the first step of starting a home health care business. It's a big decision that influences everything from the laws you'll need to follow to the qualifications of the professional caregivers and employees you hire.

There are two main types of home care agencies, each with its own benefits and limitations. The structure that's right for you all depends on how you'd like to provide services and what you want to accomplish.

22

NON-MEDICAL HOME HEALTH CARE AGENCY

Non-Medical Home Health care agencies support aging in place. Potential clients could include seniors who need some assistance around the house but otherwise are in a healthy mental state. Instead of admitting senior citizens into nursing homes, relatives can have peace of mind that their loved ones are being cared for while they remain independent.

A non-medical home health care business may only require caregivers, home care aides, or certified nursing assistants.

Services of this type of business include:

- Assisting with personal care and hygiene needs
- Prepare meals and fold laundry
- Transportation to doctors appointments
- Medication reminders
- Companionship care

When running a home care agency, potential clients may be:

- Senior citizens who need assistance with the activities of daily living (i.e., bathing, personal

- care, dressing), whether due to mobility issues or general age-related changes
- Seniors requiring transportation to and from doctors' appointments, friends' houses, stores or activities
- Elderly individuals who are isolated and can benefit from companionship
- Loved ones who need help with their caregiving responsibilities

The benefits of starting a non-medical home care business include:

- It's easier.
- While you will want to check the licensing requirements of your state or province, even if you do need a license for your agency, the regulations are much less stringent when medical care isn't being provided. You'll face fewer obstacles when setting up your business and getting proper accreditation.
- There's less overhead.
- A non-medical home care agency will have less overhead than a medical home health care business. Your professional liability insurance premiums will be lower, and you'll require fewer supplies. You also won't need to hire a clinical supervisor or licensed medical caregivers, which will keep your staffing costs lower.
- You'll be able to provide most of the necessary care.
- About 80% of the care provided by any agency is non-medical. As a home care business, you'll be

able to address the vast majority of your clients' needs and retain a large market share.

MEDICAL HOME HEALTH CARE AGENCY

The names are similar, but traditional home healthcare agencies differ from home care agencies in a few ways. While medical home health care agencies still support aging in place and independence, they also provide other services that go beyond meal preparation and personal care, requiring registered nurses and medical professionals. Regulations for this type of business are much stricter and your state may expect Medicaid certifications.

These services can include:

- Nursing care
- Blood pressure checks
- Wound care
- Occupational therapy
- Palliative care
- Physical therapy

Typical clients of a medical home care agency include:

- Seniors who have significant or chronic medical conditions
- Senior citizens who were recently discharged

from a hospital, rehab or skilled nursing facility but need additional care
- Terminally ill individuals who wish to spend their final days at home
- Seniors who need monitoring after a recent injury or medication change
- People who are not healthy enough to safely travel to a doctor's office
- Seniors who have had a decline in function and require help to regain independence

A lot goes into establishing a health care business. To set up your business successfully, you need to be aware of all of the legal information, licensing requirements, and insurance recommendations.

Benefits of Starting a Medical Home Care Business

You'll have a one-stop-shop.

A medical home care business is able to offer full-spectrum care. You can provide a much larger array of services that go beyond assistance with daily activities to include skilled nursing, wound care, palliative care, and more. Having overlapping medical and non-medical services will expand your client base and create more revenue streams.

Ensures better retention

As clients age, their needs often change. As a medical home health care business, your services can evolve with each client, and you won't risk losing them when something medical pops up.

Helps you get your foot in the door

Many people choose in-home care as a temporary measure after a relative is discharged from the hospital, say, for example, after having surgery.

A professional from a medical home health care agency comes in and helps with things like administering medication, supporting rehabilitation, and light housework while the client recovers. This lets you develop relationships with these clients and their families, expanding your network and increasing the likelihood they'll call you down the road if long-term assistance is needed.

Gives you peace of mind

Even seniors who are relatively healthy can experience a medical emergency. With licensed medical professionals on your staff, you'll have peace of mind knowing they'll be able to handle any and all scenarios professionally and safely.

EASY STEPS TO START YOUR OWN HOME CARE BUSINESS

Once you've decided to go ahead and start offering home care services for seniors, you'll need to do the following:

Come up with a business plan

A successful business doesn't just happen overnight. Once you've come up with the idea, you'll need to create a basic business strategy that addresses what you need to turn a profit and how you'll get there. As an entrepreneur, your business plan should help you better respond to opportunities in order to succeed.

Pick your services

The extent of your home care services will depend on several factors, including your budget. As a cheaper alternative to the treatment you'd typically receive in a hospital, this could influence the extent of services or products you choose to offer. Providing wound care and injections, for example, will cost much less than purchasing the medical equipment needed to run chemotherapy or paying staff to perform 24-hour emergency care. There are many services, both medical and non-medical, that you can offer your clients. Some of these include:

- Skilled nursing
- Therapy (including physical therapy and massage therapy)
- Dietary planning/education
- Support monitoring
- Wound/surgical care

Give your business a name

Once you've established your client base and the services you'd like to provide, you'll need to select a name for your business. It's a good idea to also create a website for your business that lists all available contact information in a clear and legible manner.

Pick your business structure

In Canada, business owners can choose between one of five different business structures: sole proprietorship, partnership, corporation, cooperative, or non-profit. As a sole proprietor, you're the sole owner of the company and are therefore in charge of making any and all business decisions.

A partnership depends on one or more individuals to make it work —choose wisely!

If you choose to register your home care business as a corporation, you're in charge of how and when you make money, and you can seek funds from investors, which can be used to grow your business.

If you choose to operate as a cooperative, you will be running an incorporated business controlled by people with shared needs and values.

Non-profit businesses can be set up just like any other business in Canada, but the employees don't benefit from any profits the business brings in. If this is your first business venture, keep this in mind, especially if it's your goal to pay out multiple employee salaries.

Obtain all licenses/certifications

Home health care services require licensing and certifications in order to operate. If you're looking to start a retirement home, you must obtain a license for your seniors' personal care business from the Retirement Homes Regulatory Authority (RHRA) and make sure that you comply with their rules and requirements.

Long-term care homes are also subject to mandatory health inspections to ensure that seniors are receiving satisfactory care. The Government of Canada can provide you with more information on any and all licenses that you will need to start a senior care business.

Get business insurance

Both small and large businesses in Canada require business insurance before you can obtain a business license. There are multiple insurance providers to choose from, all with varying levels of coverage. After you decide on a provider, simply gather all of the necessary documents, and apply over the phone or online.

Hire employees

Running a home health care business for seniors is too much work for just one person, even if you're a people pleaser! When you work in healthcare, the people you hire are just as important as the people you help. These individuals will be taking care of your clients, and the best way to get more business referrals is from clients who feel that their needs are being met or exceeded.

While you yourself do not need to have a healthcare background, your staff should, as they'll be the ones in charge of administering medications, overseeing treatment plans, and performing medical and non-medical applications like wound care and physiotherapy. You should have at least one registered nurse on staff at all times and several personal support workers who have the required training and certifications, like CPR and standard first aid. As always, make sure to conduct a thorough criminal reference check on anybody that you hire, as they will be working for a vulnerable population and as the business owner, you're ultimately responsible for the well-being of your clients at all times.

Buy supplies

The supplies you need for your elderly home care business will depend on the kinds of services you will provide. Many wholesalers in Canada specialize in medical supplies, which is a much more cost-effective option than purchasing things on an individual basis.

It's a good idea to always have commonly used items, like disposable gloves and disinfectant on hand at all times. You can also seek out a medical products supplier or manufacturer and deal with them directly, as opposed to going the wholesale route.

Spread the word

Funding your business is essential to its success! Once you've raised enough capital and have a steady client base to start, you'll need to get the word out that you're open for business. Some of your best business could come from your current business—happy clients are likely to tell their friends, who may be in need of similar services, and those referrals are crucial! It's also a good idea to be active on social media. After setting up your website, create social media accounts and start churning out content that will resonate with the clients you're looking to attract.

Starting a homecare business for the elderly offers a long-term solution for those who are looking to receive care, but do not want to leave the comfort of their own homes.

SETTING THE PRICING STRATEGY FOR YOUR HOME CARE AGENCY

As a home care agency owner, your priorities include getting clients and discussing the responsibilities your organization will assume. The next most important thing that such individuals will want to know is how much you will charge for the services your agency will be offering. Several factors come into play, in this case, including the qualifications of your employees, the services a particular client requires, extra tasks that may increase the workload, thereby warranting an additional charge, among other things.

For that reason, there is no exact science when deciding how much you should charge clients as a home care agency operator. That is the case because you need to be mindful of one's budget and ensure that your pricing strategy is competitive at the same time.

There is also the risk of overcharging your clients or leaving money on the table, especially if you do not adopt an informed pricing strategy and when you fail to evaluate your billing rates from time to time. Here is some insight into setting the pricing strategy for your home care agency.

Consider The Level and Type of Your Care Services

Home care agency services range from simple companionship to fairly involved medical care. Indeed, the demands of a particular client and the complexity of tasks will dictate how much your home care agency should charge for the services it offers specific individuals. Also, you cannot afford to overlook a patient's medical needs and medical history, as well.

For instance, if your agency is handling individuals requiring specialized medical equipment or those with a history of stroke or patients with dementia, providing them a high level of care will be necessary. That means that the rate for such persons will be higher. You also need to factor in rate adjustments as the needs of various clients changes with time.

On the other hand, if your home care agency deals with couples rather than individuals on various occasions, you may need to charge extra depending on the care level that such persons demand.

Research The Average Rates within Your Locality

Although there are many variations from one area to the next, home health aides in the U.S. charge a median of $23 per hour, according to a survey by Genworth. Of course, you do not expect the price of a gallon of milk or the cost of renting an apartment to be the same everywhere, and in the same way, agencies working with more qualified caregivers will charge more for their services.

Rate fluctuations in the case of home care agencies depend

on various factors, including locality. As such, you need to find out what other home care agency owners within your area are charging their clients to gain insight into what your pricing strategy should be. After that, you can adjust your rate upwards or downwards depending on your workers' experience and the responsibilities they undertake.

Focus on Benefits and Compensation

Sometimes, what your home care agency opts to charge clients on an hourly basis may not be the only way you compensate your caregivers for the services they provide. As such, you may find that some families are willing to give perks over and above the standard pay rate of your agency. Some of these benefits and compensation include;

- Contributions toward health insurance premiums.
- Paid time off.
- Overtime pay.
- Annual bonuses.

Working with clients who offer such benefits and compensation means that there will be an adjustment on the rates your home care agency offers.

Factor in The Skills and Experience of Your Employees

As is the case in other industries, caregivers with more education and experience will charge more for their services. The fact that some seniors require advanced care implies that your home care agency needs someone with special licenses or certifications to handle such patients. For that reason, the services that such staff members offer will cost more, and you need to consider that when setting your pricing strategy.

Some of the qualifications that may require you to pay particular caregivers more include;

- Certified Patient Care Tech (PCTs).
- Registered nurses.
- Certified Nursing Assistants (CNAs).

If your home care agency works with some employees whose services warrant higher pay, you will need to pass on the cost to clients requiring the services of professionals.

What Should Your Agency Charge for Extra Services?

Every situation and family your home care agency handles may be different. Still, the rate you charge should generally cover all essential tasks that allow your clients to live comfortably, including light housekeeping, preparing meals, running errands, managing medications, and offering assistance while bathing.

Should some of your clients ask an employee to take on additional responsibilities beyond the basic services, you need to charge extra for such tasks. Below are examples of the other services a client may require.

- Transportation using a caregiver's vehicle.
- Caring for pets.
- Accompanying a client to special events or traveling with them on trips.

The inconvenience, norm, or additional workload should dictate your home care agency charges for these extra services.

WHEN TO REVIEW YOUR PRICING

Discussing rate adjustments with your clients ahead of time is critical. The reason is that some seniors rarely consider pricing reviews, yet they are necessary because they allow your home care agency to meet various financial obligations. In that case, you need to ensure that clients factor in a schedule of rate reviews in the initial agreement, and that may include a minimum annual increase in charges.

Note that establishing a range instead of a fixed amount for rate adjustments allows your clients to increase what they pay in line with your employees' performance.

TIPS FOR HOW TO GET CLIENTS

Whether you are just starting your home care business or looking to expand your existing business, gaining clients is an important key to success. You likely know this but might be uncertain of how to get clients and where to even begin.

Learning how to get clients for private duty home care is as simple as following these tips.

CREATE A STRATEGY

It's imperative that you have a strategy for marketing. Otherwise, any move you make will be a shot in the dark. It's similar to shooting an arrow blindfolded with no idea where the target is located.

This may lead to some growth, but it more often leads to a lot of hard work going to waste. When you take the time to create a clearly defined strategy, however, you can take a much more targeted approach.

You need to be clear, first and foremost, on who you want to target. From that, you can research to determine the types of marketing materials you need and where you need to focus your efforts.

By planning each step as much as possible, you take out a lot of the guesswork and aim your arrows in the right direction.

PROVIDE GREAT CARE

All of your marketing efforts will be for nothing if you do not provide great care to patients. Word of mouth always has and always will be one of the best ways to make or break a business.

From the first point of contact to every subsequent interaction with your clients, you should treat them with the best care possible. This means that you will need to spend a good amount of time recruiting, hiring, and onboarding your employees. Ensure that they are prepared to provide the level and quality of care that you require.

It can also be an effective method to start a recognition program for your caregivers. A recognition program will reward those who are meeting your standards and motivate others to do the same.

PROFESSIONAL REFERRALS

Referrals are one of the most effective and most budget-friendly ways to build your client base. As stated above, word of mouth from current and previous clients is an incredible home health referral avenue. However, you also want to gain professional referrals when possible. There are a few great ways to do this.

One of the best ways is to cultivate relationships with doctors' offices in your area. As you are learning how to get clients for private duty home care, be sure not to overdo it. Start with one or two offices, as the idea is to allow them to get to know you as someone that will care for your patients. If they believe that you will do that, they will recommend you to others.

After connecting with doctors' offices, provide them with brochures to pass on to their patients. Offer your brochures to hospitals so that nurses can add them to discharge papers. Hospice care agencies can also share your brochures when a patient can benefit from your services.

VOLUNTEER

Giving back to your local community can go a long way in getting your name out and building trust. Consider activities such as the following:

- Spending time helping out at a homeless shelter or soup kitchen
- Holding a clothing drive or Christmas toy drive for needy families
- Organizing a blood drive
- Hosting a school supplies drive or another fundraiser for a school
- Organizing a park or beach clean-up, depending on where you live

Any activity you can do that helps others and puts you in front of your local market is a great idea. Consider having T-shirts made, to wear and hand out at these events, as well.

If you need help choosing a cause, connect with local schools, churches, food banks, and other organizations to determine the greatest need.

SPONSOR EVENTS

On a similar note, you can sponsor different types of events. For example, senior foot races or continuing education classes are great places to get in front of your target market.

While senior events should be a priority, don't overlook other events. Even if seniors are not present, their children and grandchildren are. Therefore, sponsoring events for younger age groups can still plant your company's name in the right people's minds.

SPEAKING ENGAGEMENTS

Consider speaking about health and aging topics at senior centers, retirement communities, assisted living facilities, and churches. Event Marketing, like speaking engagements, gives you the opportunity to educate your market, put a friendly face to your company name, and give the audience a sense of the care they would receive from you.

PARTNER WITH OTHER BUSINESSES

An excellent way to get new clients is to partner with other companies. The idea is to reciprocate referrals. When they come across someone who can benefit from your services, they refer that person to you. You do the same when you find someone who can benefit from their business.

While this can be a very effective method, it must be done with the utmost care. Every time you refer someone, your reputation is on the line. If that person or business does not meet expectations, your reputation takes a hit.

On the other hand, if that business does a great job, your reputation benefits. The same is true for your referral partners. Your company's performance impacts their reputation.

Due to the risk to your company's image, it is crucial that you be selective when choosing referral partners. Do some research on that company first to ensure that they do provide quality services.

DELEGATE AND OUTSOURCE

Building a business, earning a great reputation, and gaining clients require that you wear many hats. Even if you are great at handling each of these things, it can be a challenge to manage them all well and at the same time.

The best thing you can do for your business, your employees, your clients, and yourself is to learn to delegate and outsource some of the responsibility. Choose where you need to focus your energy, and then let others focus on the rest.

Start by determining what your current employees can take on. You do not want to take anyone's focus away from your clients, so ensure that any task you delegate does not interfere with those duties.

Provide any necessary training and set proper expectations and goals for each task. Then, you can oversee the progress without taking your focus away from other essential duties.

Some tasks, such as lead generation or appointment setting, can be outsourced to quality companies.

BE ACTIVE ONLINE

You are probably aiming to target your local senior market, but you must remember that at least a portion of your market may not be local. For example, potential patients may live nearby, but their family members might be across the country.

If a family member is looking for care for their loved one and lives elsewhere, they can only go by what they see online. Even if the potential patient mentions your company name, the family will want to research you before making any decisions.

This is why it is essential to be active online. By having a website and social media accounts, you make your company information accessible to family members all around the world.

Additionally, gathering email addresses on your website and social accounts opens another marketing door. You can send out email marketing campaigns that help bring in even more business.

Managing your online presence and email marketing can be time-consuming, so it's important that this be a task you either delegate to others or obtain the tools for.

You can also choose from several automated social media schedulers or companies to help build your business.

TRACK YOUR EFFORTS

Set up a tracking system to help you determine where each potential patient is coming from. By connecting your different marketing strategies, such as your website or social media accounts, you can generate marketing reports that provide details about which marking campaigns brought in the most patients. These insights will allow you to focus on the marketing efforts that are bringing in the most customers and target even more potential clients.

MANAGEMENT TIPS

Starting a private non-medical home care business is a tough but rewarding venture. The growth outlook for home care agencies is strong, but the work is demanding.

TIPS RELATED TO OFFICE/ ADMIN STAFF – THE BACKBONE OF YOUR HOME CARE BUSINESS

Recognize that your office staff are one of the single biggest factors in the success or failure of your new home care agency. Hire accordingly, and be particularly careful about hiring friends or family members; it can be difficult to know who will be a good fit for your agency long-term, and you don't want to set yourself up to have to choose between business success and personal relationships.

Don't delay establishing accountability systems for your staff. Identify 1-2 metrics that measure the most important output of each role, work with each team member to set a realistic weekly goal for their metric, and hold them accountable to hitting that goal. We list some suggested metrics in the third section of this article.

Hire a scheduler who likes solving tough puzzles. Caregivers with full-time hours that fit their schedule rarely quit—so a scheduler who can solve the Rubik's cube of good scheduling is someone to find and hang on to.

Hire for new staff positions before the need becomes urgent. If you wait to hire until you're desperate, you're much more likely to make a subpar hire. Additionally, they might be starting in circumstances where they have less time to train as well as more problems to deal with from day 1.

Understand that every single interaction with your agency shapes people's perception of your brand, not just caregiver visits. Every conversation, every visit, and every phone call help to make or break your brand.

Recognize that as your business grows, it will grow its own culture whether you intend it or not. Your choice is simply whether or not to be deliberate about what kind of culture grows.

Give your employees the benefit of the doubt, but don't make excuses to keep someone you know is a poor fit. It makes your life harder and does them a disservice.

Wherever possible, learn to measure your staff's performance on output, not input. The results they drive matter more than the time they put in. This is especially true if they're working remotely.

From your very first hires, your eventual goal should be to build a team that can operate without you. While that goal is years away, the more you keep it focus at the beginning, the more you'll gravitate toward hiring the people who will make your life easier long-term.

TIPS RELATED TO RECRUITING, RETAINING, AND MANAGING CAREGIVERS

Learn your caregivers' birthdays and text them on their birthdays. It's a small gesture that goes a long way, and they'll love you for it.

As you're implementing training, use a blended solution for caregiver training (a mix of both online and in-person trainings). We survey thousands of caregivers every month about their experiences, and demand for blended learning formats is a topic that comes up constantly.

Treat your caregivers the way you want them to treat your clients. In the course of starting a private home care business it's easy to get so caught up in business operations that you don't take an interest in your individual caregivers. Your treatment of them will determine their treatment of your clients to a large extent.

When a caregiver applies to your agency, get them in for an interview as soon as possible—same-day or next-day if possible. If they seem like a good fit, get them to their orientation and first shift as quickly as possible. Time to first shift is usually the biggest determinant of getting caregivers to work for you (once they're in your hiring process) vs. losing them to another opportunity.

Get in the mindset that you are always recruiting. Possibly excluding the initial phase of getting your first 6-8 clients, there will be always be a need for new caregivers and it's almost impossible to get too many caregivers.

Text each new caregiver before their first shift to check in and see if they have any more questions. This will help them get started on a good note and also help you avoid caregiver no-shows.

In your job postings, don't require qualifications that you could easily help them achieve in a night of training. Your agency will miss out on good applicants otherwise.

Use texting as one of your channels to communicate with caregivers. You can set up business SMS accounts for relatively cheap, and the advantage of quick, reliable communication with caregivers in their preferred channel is invaluable.

Resist the temptation to view caregivers as replaceable commodities. They are priceless assets.

TIPS RELATED TO PROVIDING GOOD CLIENT CARE

You or a member of your staff (not the regular caregiver) should call every client regularly just to check up on them. Multiple channels of communication are important, and it sends a good message about your agency cares when someone in a management position calls to see how everything is going.

Start a system to keep a pulse on how visits are going. On a similar note, you should establish channels where clients (and employees) can give feedback if they're the kind of people who are normally reluctant to do so. Caregivers will make mistakes, and that's fine as long as you know about them and can take steps to address them. Early on, it'll be easy to know exactly how every client is doing, but as your business scales you'll need to come up with deliberate processes to get regular feedback from your clients or mistakes will start to slip through the cracks.

In a service business, nothing is more important than perfecting the experience you provide to your clients. Keep a laser focus on client experience.

Hire caregivers who are good communicators and have

warm personalities. It makes a huge difference to the clients in their care.

TIPS RELATED TO YOUR OWN LEADERSHIP, TIME MANAGEMENT, AND SELF-CARE

Find mentors who can help you. Even Tiger Woods has a coach.

Study servant leadership. Servant leadership is a particularly important leadership style for someone starting a home care agency; it will shape the entire culture of your business to care about people.

Get enough sleep. Starting and running a home care agency takes energy.

Schedule regular 'clarity breaks' to work on the business instead of in the business. If you don't think big picture regularly, you'll struggle to run your business because your business will be running you.

Your home care scheduling software is your best friend —as is technology in general. Agencies that use their software properly typically operate far more efficiently.

Long-term and all else held equal, and agency that embraces the right technology will leave an agency that avoids technology in its dust.

Find a community where you can talk to other agency owners, whether it's a Facebook group, membership network, franchise group, or accountability group. You'll need the support.

Read Leadership and Self-Deception by the Arbinger Institute. It will change how you view leadership and personal relationships.

TIPS TO GROW YOUR HOME CARE BUSINESS

Make sure you understand the costs and are prepared to cover them. The average amount that owners spent to start a non-medical, private duty home care agency through its first six months in 2019 was $60,000, though some reported spending as little as $9,000 and as much as $260,000. (Home Care Benchmarking Study data)

Remember that there are three ways to bring in more revenue:

- getting more clients,
- increasing per-client revenue, and
- retaining clients longer.

While the first is a necessity when you're starting out, your ability to manage the second and third will play a huge role in your profitability and growth as you scale the business. Don't neglect any of these pillars.

Invest in getting good online reviews from the start. 90% of consumers read online reviews before making a purchase, and this number is probably even higher for a major decision like in-home care.

Unless you come from a background in digital marketing, consider hiring a marketing agency to manage your website, SEO, and Google Ads. It'll take a lot of strain off you and your online presence is worth the cost of doing right.

Develop something that differentiates your agency, both to potential clients and to referral sources. Saying how great your caregivers are or are much you care isn't enough; anybody can say that. You need something specific, easily communicated, and concrete. For instance, you might train your caregivers to focus on helping clients get enough socialization and make that a key talking point in your marketing. Quality of caregivers can be a great differentiator, but you would need to go truly above and beyond with multiple other sources (client reviews, third-party awards, testimonials) to validate your claim.

Understand that establishing relationships with referral partners takes time. It takes 8-12 visits with the average referral source before you receive a single referral from them.

Use client referral programs and employee referral programs. When executed properly, they typically yield the most loyal clients and the longest-tenured caregivers. Volume of referrals will be tiny as you're starting, but the more quickly you can put these programs in place the more rapidly you can scale.

In general, plan on hiring a sales rep at around 1,000 weekly billable hours. Until then, you'll need to be thinking about how to make your referral partnerships dependent on a process, not on you as a person, so that you'll be able to successfully hand them off when the time comes.

It's almost always better to have a few solid referral

relationships than many weak ones. As you start to get online reviews, respond to every review regardless of whether it's positive or negative. If it's positive, thank them. If it's negative, give them your number and invite them to reach out to you directly. Whether or not they take you up on it, this sends a great message to other people looking at your reviews.

CHALLENGES

While the senior population is expected to increase by over 80 percent within the next 25 years, more entrepreneurs and established companies are entering the senior care industry.

Many nurses, certified nursing assistants and other caregivers are attracted to the flexibility that working in the senior care industry can provide. But companies newly entering the market are also encountering a number of challenges.

STARTUP AND ONGOING COSTS

Startup costs for a home health care, hospice or private duty care agencies can be substantial. The purchase of software management systems, vehicles, uniforms and capital equipment alone can run into the tens of thousands of dollars. Additional substantial costs includes the procurement of appropriate certifications, state and local licenses along with professional liability insurance to cover falls and other accidents in individuals' homes. Other costs include compliance with local labor laws and provision of health insurance coverage and other benefits in addition to salaries for employees.

FINDING AND KEEPING QUALITY STAFF

For new companies, marketing and advertising to recruit and train quality staff can be a major expense. But the largest expense for a home health care agency will be salaries or payments to employees. With demand for home health and private duty care increasing, many health care workers are in demand and can command competitive salaries and benefits.

In order to retain exceptional staff members, home care agencies must provide continuing education along with regular pay increases and competitive benefits packages.

CLOSING THE COMMUNICATION GAP WITH HOSPITALS AND MEDICAL PROVIDERS

In accordance with new legislation, medical providers either have moved or are in process of moving to electronic health records. The use of diagnostic devices is becoming increasingly common to connect to remote networks for digital data input. For home health, hospice and private duty care companies and workers, this means navigating an array of complex devices and systems.

Learning the new systems can take extensive time and financial investment. For small companies especially, the need to keep up with constantly changing technology can be a burden.

Confusion with "Home Care vs Home Health Care; Medical vs Non-Medical"

Significant confusion exists over the differences between

home health care and home care. Home health care is medically necessary and prescribed episodic rehabilitative treatment for short term diagnosis of illness or injuries.The care is delivered in a home setting by trained and licensed nurse or therapist as directed by a physician. Home care, also called private duty care, is not directed by a physician and must not include any type of medical care or treatment. Home care services are also delivered in a home setting and includes non-medical tasks such as assistance with ADL's (activities of daily living) for example; cooking, bathing and dressing. Some private duty home care agencies present their employees as medical professionals when they've gone through only non-standard, proprietary training programs. Retaining a licensed nurse on staff often adds to the confusion.

The muddled presentation creates confusion in the marketplace about what workers are and are not allowed to do in individual's' homes. For many home health care companies, marketing and education to help reduce the confusion represents a significant expense.

PROMISING GROWTH, DAUNTING CHALLENGES

Despite the lure of significant potential growth in the coming years, the senior care industry also faces a number of challenges. Along with startup and ongoing costs, a steep technology learning curve, confusion in the marketplace, constantly changing legislation and licensing requirements, as well as attracting and retaining quality employees will continue to be major obstacles.